OSTEOPOROSIS DIET COOKBOOK FOR WOMEN

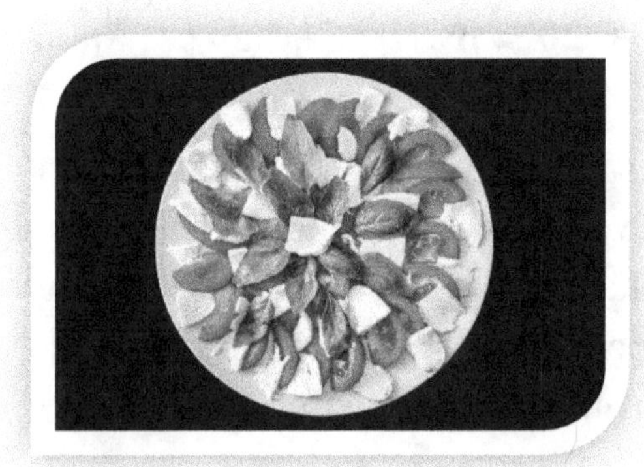

Healthy and easy nutrition guide with calcium-rich recipes for healthy joints and bones

DR.CATHERINE THOMAS

TABLE OF CONTENT

Welcome to the "Osteoporosis Diet Cookbook for Women." I'm Dr. Catherine Thomas, a nutritionist with years of experience dedicated to helping individuals achieve optimal health through proper nutrition. This book is a labor of love, inspired by both my professional journey and a deeply personal story. A few years ago, my college roommate, Sarah, was diagnosed with osteoporosis at a surprisingly young age. The news was devastating, and it felt as though a dark cloud had settled over her future. Sarah had always been vibrant and full of life, but the diagnosis threatened to take that away from her. Determined not to let the disease dictate her life, Sarah embarked on a mission to fight back with every tool at her disposal. She consulted with specialists, read countless books, and, most importantly, began to explore the powerful impact of nutrition. Together, we delved into the world of anti-inflammatory diets, discovering foods that could help strengthen her bones and reduce inflammation. We experimented with various ingredients, tested recipes, and adjusted our diets to support her health goals. It was a journey of learning, perseverance, and hope. As Sarah's condition began to improve, it became clear that the right diet could make a significant difference in managing and even reversing the effects of osteoporosis. Her transformation was nothing short of miraculous. She regained her strength, her energy levels soared, and she reclaimed her life. Inspired by Sarah's success and driven by my passion for nutrition, I decided to compile our knowledge and experiences into this cookbook. My goal is to provide you with a comprehensive guide filled with nutritious and flavorful anti-inflammatory recipes designed to naturally combat osteoporosis and enhance your overall health.

In these pages, you'll find a variety of recipes that are not only delicious but also packed with essential nutrients to support bone health. From hearty breakfasts to satisfying dinners, each recipe has been carefully crafted to help you on your journey towards stronger bones and a healthier lifestyle. I invite you to join me on this culinary adventure.

Let's embrace the power of nutrition together and discover how the right diet can transform your life, just as it did for Sarah. Here's to stronger bones, better health, and a brighter future.

Warm regards,

Dr. Catherine Thomas

CHAPTER 1

Understanding Osteoporosis

Osteoporosis is a progressive bone disease characterized by decreased bone density and mass, leading to fragile bones and an increased risk of fractures. It is often referred to as the "silent disease" because it progresses without symptoms until a fracture occurs. Osteoporosis primarily affects older adults, with a higher prevalence in women, particularly postmenopausal women.

Types of Osteoporosis

1. **Primary Osteoporosis:**

    Type I (Postmenopausal Osteoporosis): This type occurs in women after menopause due to a significant drop in estrogen levels. Estrogen plays a crucial role in maintaining bone density, and its deficiency accelerates bone loss.

    Type I osteoporosis commonly affects trabecular bone, which is found in the spine, hips, and wrists.

Type II (Senile Osteoporosis): This type affects both men and women over the age of 70. It results from the natural aging process, where bone formation decreases, and bone resorption increases. Senile osteoporosis affects both cortical and trabecular bones, leading to fractures in the hips, vertebrae, and long bones.

2. **Secondary Osteoporosis**: This form of osteoporosis is caused by other medical conditions or medications that affect bone metabolism. Conditions such as hyperthyroidism, chronic kidney disease, rheumatoid arthritis, and the use of glucocorticoids can lead to secondary osteoporosis. Addressing the underlying condition is crucial for managing this type of osteoporosis.

Causes of Osteoporosis

Osteoporosis occurs when the balance between bone formation and bone resorption is disrupted. Several factors contribute to this imbalance:

1. **Hormonal Changes**: In women, decreased estrogen levels after menopause accelerate bone loss. In men, a decline in testosterone levels with age can also affect bone density.

2. **Calcium and Vitamin D Deficiency**: Calcium and vitamin D are essential for bone health.

3. Inadequate intake or absorption of these nutrients can lead to weakened bones.

4. **Age**: Bone density peaks in early adulthood and gradually decreases with age. The risk of osteoporosis increases significantly after the age of 50.

5. **Genetics**: A family history of osteoporosis or fractures can increase the likelihood of developing the disease.

6. **Lifestyle Factors**:

     Sedentary Lifestyle: Lack of physical activity, especially weight-bearing exercises, can lead to bone loss.

     Smoking: Smoking has a negative impact on bone health and can reduce bone density.

     Alcohol Consumption: Excessive alcohol intake can interfere with calcium absorption and bone formation.

7. **Medications**: Long-term use of certain medications, such as glucocorticoids, anticonvulsants, and proton pump inhibitors, can affect bone density.

Symptoms of Osteoporosis

Osteoporosis is often called the "silent disease" because it develops slowly over many years without any noticeable symptoms. However,

once bones have been significantly weakened, symptoms may include:

1. Fractures: The most common and serious complication of osteoporosis is fractures.

   These can occur with minimal trauma or even spontaneously. Common fracture sites include the hip, spine, and wrist.

2. Back Pain: Compression fractures of the vertebrae can cause severe back pain, often leading to a hunched posture known as kyphosis or "dowager's hump."

3. Loss of Height: Vertebral fractures can cause a loss of height over time.

4. Bone Pain: In advanced stages, patients may experience bone pain and tenderness.

Preventive Measures for Osteoporosis

Preventing osteoporosis involves a combination of lifestyle changes, dietary modifications, and, in some cases, medications. Here are some key strategies:

1. **Adequate Calcium Intake**: Ensure sufficient calcium intake through diet or supplements. Good dietary sources of calcium include dairy products, leafy green vegetables, fortified foods, and fish with edible bones. The recommended daily intake of calcium varies by age and sex but generally ranges from 1,000 to 1,300 mg per day.

2. **Sufficient Vitamin D**: Vitamin D is crucial for calcium absorption and bone health. Sun exposure helps the body produce vitamin D, but dietary sources and supplements are often necessary, especially in regions with limited sunlight. The recommended daily intake of vitamin D is about 600 to 800 IU, depending on age and risk factors.

3. **Regular Exercise**: Engage in weight-bearing exercises, such as walking, jogging, dancing, and strength training. These activities help build and maintain bone density. Balance and flexibility exercises, such as yoga and tai chi, can reduce the risk of falls and fractures.

4. **Healthy Diet**: A balanced diet rich in fruits, vegetables, lean proteins, and whole grains supports overall health and provides essential nutrients for bone health. Avoid excessive caffeine and salt, as they can negatively impact bone density.

5. **Avoid Smoking and Limit Alcohol**: Smoking cessation and moderation of alcohol intake are critical for maintaining bone health. Smoking decreases bone mass, while excessive alcohol consumption interferes with calcium absorption and bone formation.

6. **Medications**: For those at high risk of fractures, medications may be prescribed to strengthen bones and reduce the risk of fractures. These can include bisphosphonates, hormone replacement therapy, selective estrogen receptor modulators (SERMs), and others. It is essential to discuss the benefits and risks of these medications with a healthcare provider.

7. **Bone Density Testing**: Regular bone density tests (DEXA scans) can help detect osteoporosis early, allowing for timely intervention. Women over the age of 65 and men over the age of 70, as well as younger individuals with risk factors, should consider getting screened.

Osteoporosis is a serious condition that can significantly impact quality of life. Understanding the causes, recognizing the symptoms, and implementing preventive measures can help manage and reduce the risk of osteoporosis. By maintaining a healthy lifestyle, ensuring adequate intake of calcium and vitamin D, and engaging in regular physical activity, individuals can protect their bone health and enhance their overall well-being.

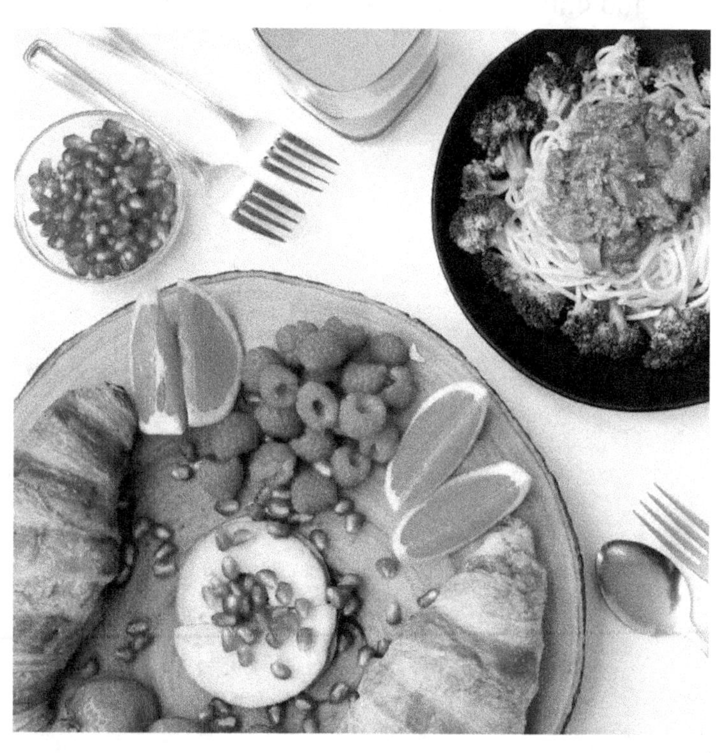

CHAPTER 2

Benefit of Osteoporosis Diet for Women

Core Benefits of Following an Osteoporosis Diet for Women

1. **Improved Bone Density**:
   Increased Calcium Intake: A diet rich in calcium from dairy products, leafy greens, and fortified foods helps build and maintain strong bones. This is crucial for women, especially postmenopausal women, who are at higher risk of bone density loss.
   Vitamin D: Adequate vitamin D levels enhance calcium absorption in the gut, ensuring that the calcium consumed is effectively used to strengthen bones.

2. **Reduced Risk of Fractures**:
   Stronger Bones: By consuming essential nutrients like calcium, vitamin D, magnesium, and vitamin K, women can improve their bone strength and reduce the likelihood of fractures, particularly in the hips, spine, and wrists.
   Muscle Health: Adequate protein intake supports muscle health, which in turn helps stabilize and protect bones, reducing the risk of falls and subsequent fractures.

3. **Anti-Inflammatory Benefits:**

Reduced Inflammation: An osteoporosis diet often includes anti-inflammatory foods such as fruits, vegetables, fatty fish, and nuts. These foods can help reduce inflammation in the body, which is beneficial for overall bone health and can alleviate symptoms in conditions associated with osteoporosis.

4. **Enhanced Nutrient Absorption:**

Balanced Diet: A well-rounded osteoporosis diet ensures that women receive a variety of nutrients essential for bone health, including calcium, vitamin D, magnesium, and vitamin K. This holistic approach promotes better overall nutrient absorption and utilization.

Healthy Gut: Including foods that promote gut health, such as probiotics from yogurt and fiber from fruits and vegetables, can improve nutrient absorption and overall digestive health.

5. **Hormonal Balance:**

Phytoestrogens: Certain foods, such as soy products, contain phytoestrogens, which can mimic the effects of estrogen in the body.

This is particularly beneficial for postmenopausal women, as estrogen helps maintain bone density.

Hormonal Health: A balanced diet that includes healthy fats and proteins can support hormonal health, which is crucial for bone maintenance.

6. **Weight Management:**

Healthy Weight: Maintaining a healthy weight is important for bone health. Excess weight can put additional stress on bones, while being underweight can lead to decreased bone density. A balanced osteoporosis diet can help women achieve and maintain a healthy weight.

Nutrient-Dense Foods: Focusing on nutrient-dense foods helps women feel full and satisfied, reducing the likelihood of overeating and weight gain.

7. **Improved Overall Health:**

Heart Health: Many foods beneficial for bone health, such as fatty fish, nuts, and leafy greens, also support cardiovascular health. Reducing sodium intake and limiting processed foods can also benefit heart health.

Mental Well-being: A nutritious diet can improve mood and cognitive function, enhancing overall quality of life.

Proper nutrition supports brain health and can reduce the risk of depression and anxiety, which are common in individuals dealing with chronic health conditions.

8. **Prevention of Other Health Issues:**

Reduced Risk of Chronic Diseases: A diet rich in fruits, vegetables, lean proteins, and whole grains can help prevent other chronic diseases such as diabetes, hypertension, and certain cancers. These conditions can complicate osteoporosis management, so preventing them is beneficial for overall health.

Enhanced Immune Function: Nutrient-rich foods support a healthy immune system, helping the body fight off infections and illnesses that could further weaken bones.

9. **Longevity and Quality of Life:**

Increased Longevity: By reducing the risk of fractures and other osteoporosis-related complications, a proper diet can contribute to a longer, healthier life.

Enhanced Mobility: Stronger bones and muscles support better mobility and independence, improving the overall quality of life for women as they age.

Foods to Eat and Avoid for Optimum Bone Health in Osteoporosis

Foods to Eat

1. **Calcium-Rich Foods:**

   Dairy Products: Milk, yogurt, and cheese are excellent sources of calcium, essential for bone health.

   Leafy Greens: Kale, collard greens, broccoli, and bok choy provide significant amounts of calcium.

   Fortified Foods: Some cereals, orange juice, and plant-based milks (like almond or soy milk) are fortified with calcium.

2. **Vitamin D Sources:**

   Fatty Fish: Salmon, mackerel, and sardines are rich in vitamin D, which helps in calcium absorption.

   Egg Yolks: Another good source of vitamin D.

Fortified Foods: Similar to calcium, many foods are fortified with vitamin D, such as milk, orange juice, and cereals.

3. **Magnesium-Rich Foods**:

Nuts and Seeds: Almonds, cashews, pumpkin seeds, and sunflower seeds.

Whole Grains: Brown rice, quinoa, and whole wheat products.

Legumes: Black beans, chickpeas, and lentils.

4. **Vitamin K Sources**:

Leafy Greens: Spinach, kale, and Swiss chard.

Cruciferous Vegetables: Brussels sprouts and broccoli.

5. **Protein-Rich Foods**:

Lean Meats: Chicken, turkey, and lean cuts of beef.

Fish: Besides being a good source of vitamin D, fish provides high-quality protein.

Plant-Based Proteins: Beans, lentils, tofu, and tempeh.

6. **Other Beneficial Foods:**

Fruits and Vegetables: Rich in vitamins, minerals, and antioxidants that support overall health.

Herbs and Spices: Turmeric and ginger have anti-inflammatory properties that can be beneficial.

Foods to Avoid

1. **High-Sodium Foods:**

Processed Foods: Packaged snacks, canned soups, and processed meats often contain high levels of sodium, which can increase calcium loss through urine.

Fast Food: Often high in both sodium and unhealthy fats.

2. **Excessive Caffeine:**

Coffee: Limit to 1-2 cups per day as excessive caffeine can interfere with calcium absorption.

Soda and Energy Drinks: These often contain high caffeine levels and phosphates that can affect bone health.

3. **Sugary Foods and Beverages**:

Sugary Snacks and Sodas: High sugar intake can lead to increased calcium excretion in the urine.

Refined Carbs: Foods like white bread, pastries, and sugary cereals can contribute to poor overall diet quality.

4. **Alcohol**:

Excessive Alcohol: Can interfere with the body's ability to absorb calcium and vitamin D, weakening bones over time. Limit alcohol intake to one drink per day for women.

5. **High-Oxalate Foods** (in moderation):

Spinach and Rhubarb: Although rich in calcium, they also contain oxalates that can inhibit calcium absorption. Consume in moderation and balance with other calcium-rich foods.

6. **High-Phosphate Foods**:

> **Processed Meats**: Often contain phosphates which can interfere with calcium balance in the body.

> **Soft Drinks**: Especially colas, which contain phosphoric acid that can affect bone health.

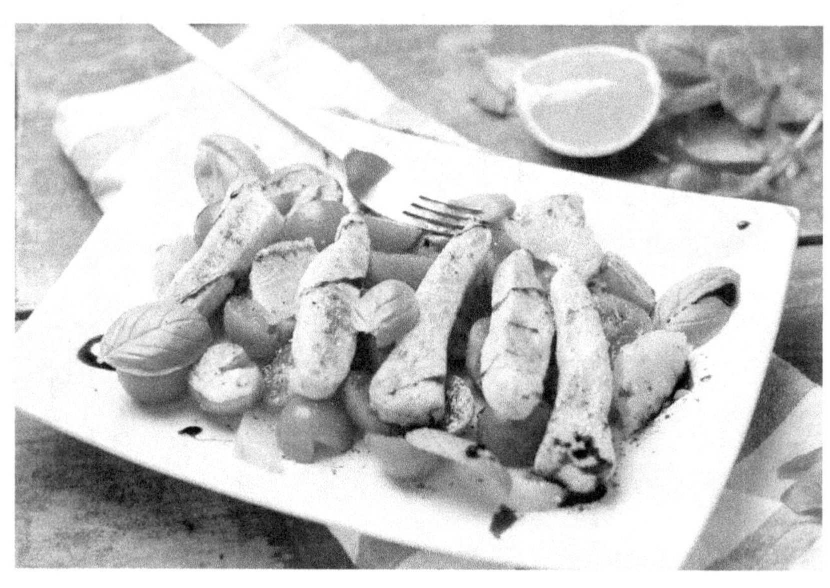

CHAPTER 3

Energizing Breakfast:

Greek Yogurt Parfait

Ingredients:

- 1 cup Greek yogurt
- 1/2 cup mixed berries (strawberries, blueberries, raspberries)
- 1/4 cup granola
- 1 tbsp honey
- 1 tbsp chia seeds

Preparation Method:

1. Layer Greek yogurt, berries, and granola in a bowl or glass.
2. Drizzle with honey.
3. Sprinkle chia seeds on top.

Cooking Time: 5 minutes

Nutritional Value (per serving):
- Calories: 300
- Protein: 15g
- Calcium: 250mg and Fiber: 6g

Spinach and Feta Omelette

Ingredients:

- 2 large eggs
- 1/2 cup fresh spinach
- 1/4 cup crumbled feta cheese
- 1 tbsp olive oil
- Salt and pepper to taste

Preparation Method:

1. Heat olive oil in a skillet over medium heat.
2. Add spinach and cook until wilted.
3. Beat eggs, pour into the skillet, and cook until set.
4. Sprinkle feta cheese, fold the omelette, and serve.

Cooking Time: 10 minutes

Nutritional Value (per serving):
- Calories: 250
- Protein: 15g
- Calcium: 200mg
- Fiber: 2g

Almond Butter Banana Toast

Ingredients:
- 1 slice whole-grain bread
- 1 tbsp almond butter
- 1/2 banana, sliced
- 1 tsp chia seeds

Preparation Method:

1. Toast the bread.
2. Spread almond butter on the toast.
3. Top with banana slices and chia seeds.

Cooking Time: 5 minutes

Nutritional Value (per serving):
- Calories: 220
- Protein: 6g
- Calcium: 100mg
- Fiber: 5g

Oatmeal with Berries and Almonds

Ingredients:

- 1/2 cup rolled oats
- 1 cup almond milk
- 1/2 cup mixed berries
- 1 tbsp sliced almonds
- 1 tsp honey

Preparation Method:

1. Cook oats in almond milk over medium heat until soft.
2. Top with berries, almonds, and honey.

Cooking Time: 10 minutes

Nutritional Value (per serving):

- Calories: 250
- Protein: 7g
- Calcium: 200mg
- Fiber: 6g

Ingredients:
- 1 slice whole-grain bread
- 1/2 avocado, mashed
- 1 large egg
- 1 tsp lemon juice
- Salt and pepper to taste

Preparation Method:

1. Toast the bread.
2. Spread mashed avocado mixed with lemon juice on the toast.
3. Poach the egg and place it on top of the avocado toast.
4. Season with salt and pepper.

Cooking Time: 10 minutes

Nutritional Value (per serving):
- Calories: 280
- Protein: 10g
- Calcium: 60mg
- Fiber: 7g

Berry Smoothie

Ingredients:
- 1 cup almond milk
- 1/2 cup Greek yogurt
- 1/2 cup mixed berries (strawberries, blueberries, raspberries)
- 1 tbsp chia seeds
- 1 tsp honey

Preparation Method:

1. Blend all ingredients until smooth.
2. Serve chilled.

Cooking Time: 5 minutes

Nutritional Value (per serving):
- Calories: 200
- Protein: 8g
- Calcium: 300mg
- Fiber: 5g

Cottage Cheese with Pineapple

Ingredients:
- 1 cup cottage cheese
- 1/2 cup fresh pineapple chunks
- 1 tbsp chopped walnuts

Preparation Method:

1. Mix cottage cheese with pineapple chunks.
2. Top with chopped walnuts.

Cooking Time: 5 minutes

Nutritional Value (per serving):
- Calories: 220
- Protein: 15g
- Calcium: 150mg
- Fiber: 2g

Chia Seed Pudding

Ingredients:
- 1/4 cup chia seeds
- 1 cup almond milk
- 1 tsp honey
- 1/2 tsp vanilla extract
- 1/4 cup mixed berries

Preparation Method:

1. Mix chia seeds, almond milk, honey, and vanilla extract.
2. Refrigerate overnight.
3. Top with mixed berries before serving.

Cooking Time: 5 minutes prep + overnight chilling

Nutritional Value (per serving):
- Calories: 250
- Protein: 5g
- Calcium: 300mg
- Fiber: 10g

Apple Cinnamon Quinoa

Ingredients:
- 1/2 cup quinoa
- 1 cup almond milk
- 1/2 apple, diced
- 1 tsp cinnamon
- 1 tbsp maple syrup

Preparation Method:

1. Cook quinoa in almond milk until tender.
2. Stir in diced apple, cinnamon, and maple syrup.

Cooking Time: 15 minutes

Nutritional Value (per serving):
- Calories: 270
- Protein: 7g
- Calcium: 200mg
- Fiber: 5g

Ingredients:

- 1 slice whole-grain bread
- 1/2 avocado, mashed
- 2 oz smoked salmon
- 1 tsp lemon juice
- Fresh dill for garnish

Preparation Method:

1. Toast the bread.
2. Spread mashed avocado mixed with lemon juice on the toast.
3. Top with smoked salmon and garnish with dill.

Cooking Time: 5 minutes

Nutritional Value (per serving):

- Calories: 250
- Protein: 12g
- Calcium: 50mg
- Fiber: 5g

Blueberry Almond Overnight Oats

Ingredients:

- 1/2 cup rolled oats
- 1/2 cup almond milk
- 1/4 cup Greek yogurt
- 1/4 cup blueberries
- 1 tbsp sliced almonds
- 1 tsp honey

Preparation Method:

1. Mix oats, almond milk, and Greek yogurt.
2. Refrigerate overnight.
3. Top with blueberries, almonds, and honey before serving.

Cooking Time: 5 minutes prep + overnight chilling

Nutritional Value (per serving):

- Calories: 300
- Protein: 10g
- Calcium: 200mg
- Fiber: 6g

Scrambled Tofu with Vegetables

Ingredients:

- 1/2 block firm tofu, crumbled
- 1/2 cup bell peppers, diced
- 1/4 cup onions, diced
- 1/4 cup spinach
- 1 tbsp olive oil
- 1/2 tsp turmeric
- Salt and pepper to taste

Preparation Method:

1. Heat olive oil in a skillet over medium heat.
2. Sauté onions and bell peppers until soft.
3. Add crumbled tofu and turmeric, and cook until heated through.
4. Stir in spinach and cook until wilted.
5. Season with salt and pepper.

Cooking Time: 10 minutes

Nutritional Value (per serving):
- Calories: 200
- Protein: 12g
- Calcium: 150mg
- Fiber: 3g

Sweet Potato Breakfast Bowl

Ingredients:
- 1 medium sweet potato, baked and mashed
- 1/4 cup Greek yogurt
- 1 tbsp almond butter
- 1 tbsp chia seeds
- 1 tsp honey
- 1/4 cup granola

Preparation Method:

1. Mix mashed sweet potato with Greek yogurt, almond butter, and honey.
2. Top with chia seeds and granola.

Cooking Time: 10 minutes

Nutritional Value (per serving):
- Calories: 350
- Protein: 10g
- Calcium: 200mg
- Fiber: 7g

Ingredients:
- 1 cup frozen mango chunks
- 1/2 cup Greek yogurt
- 1/2 cup almond milk
- 1 tbsp chia seeds
- 1/4 cup granola
- 1/4 cup fresh mango, diced

Preparation Method:

1. Blend frozen mango, Greek yogurt, and almond milk until smooth.
2. Pour into a bowl and top with chia seeds, granola, and fresh mango.

Cooking Time: 5 minutes

Nutritional Value (per serving):
- Calories: 300
- Protein: 10g
- Calcium: 200mg
- Fiber: 5g

Peanut Butter and Banana Smoothie

Ingredients:
- 1 cup almond milk
- 1 banana
- 2 tbsp peanut butter
- 1/4 cup Greek yogurt
- 1 tbsp chia seeds

Preparation Method:

1. Blend all ingredients until smooth.
2. Serve chilled.

Cooking Time: 5 minutes

Nutritional Value (per serving):
- Calories: 350
- Protein: 12g
- Calcium: 250mg
- Fiber: 6g

Flavorful Lunch:

Grilled Chicken Salad

Ingredients:
- 4 oz grilled chicken breast
- 2 cups mixed greens
- 1/2 cup cherry tomatoes, halved
- 1/4 cup cucumber, sliced
- 1/4 cup feta cheese, crumbled
- 1 tbsp olive oil
- 1 tbsp balsamic vinegar
- Salt and pepper to taste

Preparation Method:

1. Grill chicken breast until fully cooked, about 6-8 minutes per side.
2. Mix greens, tomatoes, cucumber, and feta cheese in a bowl.
3. Slice chicken and place on top of the salad.
4. Drizzle with olive oil and balsamic vinegar, and season with salt and pepper.

Cooking Time: 20 minutes

Nutritional Value (per serving):
- Calories: 350
- Protein: 30g
- Calcium: 200mg and Fiber: 4g

Quinoa and Black Bean Bowl

Ingredients:
- 1/2 cup quinoa, cooked
- 1/2 cup black beans, cooked
- 1/4 cup corn
- 1/2 avocado, diced
- 1/4 cup salsa
- 1 tbsp lime juice
- 1 tbsp cilantro, chopped

Preparation Method:

1. Cook quinoa according to package instructions.
2. Combine quinoa, black beans, corn, avocado, and salsa in a bowl.
3. Drizzle with lime juice and sprinkle with cilantro.

Cooking Time: 15 minutes

Nutritional Value (per serving):
- Calories: 400
- Protein: 12g
- Calcium: 60mg
- Fiber: 12g

Ingredients:

- 1 whole-grain tortilla
- 1 cup fresh spinach
- 1/2 cup mushrooms, sliced
- 1/4 cup hummus
- 1 tbsp olive oil
- Salt and pepper to taste

Preparation Method:

1. Heat olive oil in a skillet over medium heat.
2. Sauté mushrooms until tender, about 5 minutes.
3. Add spinach and cook until wilted.
4. Spread hummus on the tortilla, add the spinach and mushroom mixture, and roll up.

Cooking Time: 10 minutes

Nutritional Value (per serving):

- Calories: 300
- Protein: 10g
- Calcium: 80mg
- Fiber: 8g

Lentil and Vegetable Soup

Ingredients:

- 1 cup lentils, rinsed
- 4 cups vegetable broth
- 1 cup carrots, diced
- 1 cup celery, diced
- 1 cup onion, diced
- 2 garlic cloves, minced
- 1 tbsp olive oil
- 1 tsp thyme
- 1 tsp rosemary
- Salt and pepper to taste

Preparation Method:

1. Heat olive oil in a pot over medium heat.
2. Sauté onion, carrots, celery, and garlic until tender, about 5 minutes.
3. Add lentils, vegetable broth, thyme, and rosemary.
4. Bring to a boil, then reduce heat and simmer for 30 minutes.
5. Season with salt and pepper.

Cooking Time: 40 minutes

Nutritional Value (per serving):

- Calories: 250
- Protein: 15g ,Calcium: 80mg and Fiber: 15g

Ingredients:
- 1 can (5 oz) tuna, drained
- 1/2 avocado, diced
- 1/4 cup red onion, diced
- 1/4 cup celery, diced
- 1 tbsp Greek yogurt
- 1 tbsp lemon juice
- Salt and pepper to taste

Preparation Method:

1. In a bowl, combine tuna, avocado, red onion, and celery.
2. Mix in Greek yogurt and lemon juice.
3. Season with salt and pepper.

Cooking Time: 10 minutes

Nutritional Value (per serving):
- Calories: 250
- Protein: 25g
- Calcium: 40mg
- Fiber: 6g

Ingredients:
- 1 cup chickpeas, cooked
- 1 cup cherry tomatoes, halved
- 1/4 cup red onion, diced
- 1/4 cup feta cheese, crumbled
- 1 tbsp olive oil
- 1 tbsp lemon juice
- 1 tbsp parsley, chopped
- Salt and pepper to taste

Preparation Method:

1. Combine chickpeas, tomatoes, red onion, and feta cheese in a bowl.
2. Drizzle with olive oil and lemon juice.
3. Sprinkle with parsley and season with salt and pepper.

Cooking Time: 10 minutes

Nutritional Value (per serving):
- Calories: 300
- Protein: 12g
- Calcium: 150mg
- Fiber: 10g

Ingredients:

- 4 oz salmon fillet
- 1 cup asparagus, trimmed
- 1 tbsp olive oil
- 1 tbsp lemon juice
- Salt and pepper to taste

Preparation Method:

1. Preheat grill to medium-high heat.
2. Drizzle salmon and asparagus with olive oil and lemon juice.
3. Season with salt and pepper.
4. Grill salmon for 4-5 minutes per side.
5. Grill asparagus for 3-4 minutes, turning occasionally.

Cooking Time: 15 minutes

Nutritional Value (per serving):

- Calories: 350
- Protein: 25g
- Calcium: 60mg
- Fiber: 4g

Turkey and Avocado Wrap

Ingredients:
- 1 whole-grain tortilla
- 4 oz sliced turkey breast
- 1/2 avocado, sliced
- 1/4 cup spinach
- 1 tbsp hummus

Preparation Method:

1. Spread hummus on the tortilla.
2. Add turkey, avocado, and spinach.
3. Roll up and slice in half.

Cooking Time: 5 minutes

Nutritional Value (per serving):
- Calories: 350
- Protein: 25g
- Calcium: 40mg
- Fiber: 8g

Ingredients:
- 1/2 cup quinoa, cooked
- 1/2 cup cherry tomatoes, halved
- 1/4 cup cucumber, diced
- 1/4 cup red onion, diced
- 1/4 cup feta cheese, crumbled
- 1 tbsp olive oil
- 1 tbsp lemon juice
- 1 tbsp oregano
- Salt and pepper to taste

Preparation Method:

1. Combine quinoa, tomatoes, cucumber, red onion, and feta in a bowl.
2. Drizzle with olive oil and lemon juice.
3. Sprinkle with oregano and season with salt and pepper.

Cooking Time: 15 minutes

Nutritional Value (per serving):
- Calories: 350
- Protein: 12g
- Calcium: 150mg
- Fiber: 6g

Stuffed Bell Peppers

Ingredients:
- 2 bell peppers, halved and seeded
- 1/2 cup quinoa, cooked
- 1/2 cup black beans, cooked
- 1/4 cup corn
- 1/4 cup salsa
- 1/4 cup shredded cheese
- 1 tbsp olive oil
- Salt and pepper to taste

Preparation Method:

1. Preheat oven to 375°F (190°C).
2. Mix quinoa, black beans, corn, and salsa.
3. Stuff bell pepper halves with the mixture.
4. Drizzle with olive oil and top with shredded cheese.
5. Bake for 20 minutes.

Cooking Time: 30 minutes

Nutritional Value (per serving):
- Calories: 300
- Protein: 12g
- Calcium: 100mg
- Fiber: 8g

Ingredients:

- 4 oz chicken breast, sliced
- 1 cup broccoli florets
- 1/2 cup bell peppers, sliced
- 1/2 cup snap peas
- 1 tbsp soy sauce
- 1 tbsp olive oil
- 1 garlic clove, minced
- 1 tsp ginger, minced

Preparation Method:

1. Heat olive oil in a skillet over medium-high heat.
2. Add garlic and ginger, sauté for 1 minute.
3. Add chicken and cook until browned, about 5-7 minutes.
4. Add vegetables and soy sauce, and stir-fry until tender, about 5 minutes.

Cooking Time: 15 minutes

Nutritional Value (per serving):

- Calories: 300
- Protein: 30g
- Calcium: 60mg
- Fiber: 5g

Spinach and Goat Cheese Stuffed Chicken

Ingredients:
- 4 oz chicken breast, butterflied
- 1 cup spinach, wilted
- 1/4 cup goat cheese, crumbled
- 1 tbsp olive oil
- Salt and pepper to taste

Preparation Method:

1. Preheat oven to 375°F (190°C).
2. Stuff chicken breast with spinach and goat cheese.
3. Secure with toothpicks and season with salt and pepper.
4. Heat olive oil in a skillet over medium-high heat, brown chicken on both sides.
5. Transfer to oven and bake for 20 minutes.

Cooking Time: 30 minutes

Nutritional Value (per serving):
- Calories: 350
- Protein: 30g
- Calcium: 150mg
- Fiber: 2g

Shrimp and Avocado Salad

Ingredients:

- 4 oz shrimp, cooked and peeled
- 2 cups mixed greens
- 1/2 avocado, diced
- 1/4 cup cherry tomatoes, halved
- 1 tbsp olive oil
- 1 tbsp lime juice
- Salt and pepper to taste

Preparation Method:

1. Combine shrimp, mixed greens, avocado, and cherry tomatoes in a bowl.
2. Drizzle with olive oil and lime juice.
3. Season with salt and pepper.

Cooking Time: 10 minutes

Nutritional Value (per serving):

- Calories: 300
- Protein: 20g
- Calcium: 100mg
- Fiber: 5g

Sweet Potato and Black Bean Tacos

Ingredients:
- 1 medium sweet potato, diced
- 1/2 cup black beans, cooked
- 1/4 cup corn
- 1/4 cup salsa
- 2 small whole-grain tortillas
- 1 tbsp olive oil
- 1 tbsp lime juice
- Salt and pepper to taste

Preparation Method:

1. Preheat oven to 400°F (200°C).
2. Toss sweet potato with olive oil, salt, and pepper, and roast for 20 minutes.
3. Warm tortillas, fill with sweet potato, black beans, corn, and salsa.
4. Drizzle with lime juice.

Cooking Time: 25 minutes

Nutritional Value (per serving):
- Calories: 350
- Protein: 10g
- Calcium: 80mg
- Fiber: 10g

Caprese Quinoa Salad

Ingredients:
- 1/2 cup quinoa, cooked
- 1/2 cup cherry tomatoes, halved
- 1/4 cup fresh mozzarella, diced
- 1/4 cup fresh basil, chopped
- 1 tbsp olive oil
- 1 tbsp balsamic vinegar
- Salt and pepper to taste

Preparation Method:

1. Combine quinoa, tomatoes, mozzarella, and basil in a bowl.
2. Drizzle with olive oil and balsamic vinegar.
3. Season with salt and pepper.

Cooking Time: 15 minutes

Nutritional Value (per serving):
- Calories: 350
- Protein: 12g
- Calcium: 150mg
- Fiber: 4g

Joyful Dinner:

Baked Lemon Herb Salmon

Ingredients:
- 4 oz salmon fillet
- 1 tbsp olive oil
- 1 tbsp lemon juice
- 1 tsp dried dill
- 1 tsp garlic powder
- Salt and pepper to taste

Preparation Method:

1. Preheat oven to 375°F (190°C).
2. Place salmon on a baking sheet.
3. Drizzle with olive oil and lemon juice.
4. Sprinkle with dill, garlic powder, salt, and pepper.
5. Bake for 15-20 minutes.

Cooking Time: 20 minutes

Nutritional Value (per serving):
- Calories: 300
- Protein: 25g
- Calcium: 30mg
- Fiber: 0g

Quinoa Stuffed Bell Peppers

Ingredients:

- 2 bell peppers, halved and seeded
- 1 cup quinoa, cooked
- 1/2 cup black beans, cooked
- 1/2 cup corn
- 1/2 cup diced tomatoes
- 1/4 cup shredded cheese
- 1 tbsp olive oil
- Salt and pepper to taste

Preparation Method:

1. Preheat oven to 375°F (190°C).
2. Mix quinoa, black beans, corn, and tomatoes.
3. Stuff bell pepper halves with the mixture.
4. Drizzle with olive oil and top with shredded cheese.
5. Bake for 25 minutes.

Cooking Time: 30 minutes

Nutritional Value (per serving):

- Calories: 350
- Protein: 12g
- Calcium: 100mg
- Fiber: 8g

Chicken and Vegetable Stir-Fry

Ingredients:

- 4 oz chicken breast, sliced
- 1 cup broccoli florets
- 1/2 cup bell peppers, sliced
- 1/2 cup snap peas
- 1 tbsp soy sauce
- 1 tbsp olive oil
- 1 garlic clove, minced
- 1 tsp ginger, minced

Preparation Method:

1. Heat olive oil in a skillet over medium-high heat.
2. Add garlic and ginger, sauté for 1 minute.
3. Add chicken and cook until browned, about 5-7 minutes.
4. Add vegetables and soy sauce, and stir-fry until tender, about 5 minutes.

Cooking Time: 15 minutes

Nutritional Value (per serving):

- Calories: 300
- Protein: 30g
- Calcium: 60mg
- Fiber: 5g

Spinach and Mushroom Stuffed Chicken

Ingredients:

- 4 oz chicken breast, butterflied
- 1 cup spinach, wilted
- 1/4 cup mushrooms, sliced
- 1/4 cup goat cheese, crumbled
- 1 tbsp olive oil
- Salt and pepper to taste

Preparation Method:

1. Preheat oven to 375°F (190°C).
2. Stuff chicken breast with spinach, mushrooms, and goat cheese.
3. Secure with toothpicks and season with salt and pepper.
4. Heat olive oil in a skillet over medium-high heat, brown chicken on both sides.
5. Transfer to oven and bake for 20 minutes.

Cooking Time: 30 minutes

Nutritional Value (per serving):

- Calories: 350
- Protein: 30g
- Calcium: 150mg
- Fiber: 2g

Shrimp and Asparagus Skillet

Ingredients:

- 4 oz shrimp, peeled and deveined
- 1 cup asparagus, trimmed
- 1 tbsp olive oil
- 1 garlic clove, minced
- 1 tbsp lemon juice
- Salt and pepper to taste

Preparation Method:

1. Heat olive oil in a skillet over medium heat.
2. Add garlic and cook for 1 minute.
3. Add shrimp and asparagus, cook until shrimp is pink and asparagus is tender, about 5-7 minutes.
4. Drizzle with lemon juice and season with salt and pepper.

Cooking Time: 10 minutes

Nutritional Value (per serving):

- Calories: 200
- Protein: 20g
- Calcium: 100mg
- Fiber: 4g

Turkey Meatballs with Zucchini Noodles

Ingredients:

- 1 lb ground turkey
- 1/4 cup breadcrumbs
- 1/4 cup Parmesan cheese, grated
- 1 egg
- 2 garlic cloves, minced
- 1 tsp Italian seasoning
- 2 zucchini, spiralized
- 1 tbsp olive oil
- Salt and pepper to taste

Preparation Method:

1. Preheat oven to 375°F (190°C).
2. Mix ground turkey, breadcrumbs, Parmesan, egg, garlic, and Italian seasoning.
3. Form into meatballs and place on a baking sheet.
4. Bake for 20 minutes.
5. Heat olive oil in a skillet, sauté zucchini noodles until tender, about 5 minutes.
6. Serve meatballs over zucchini noodles.

Cooking Time: 30 minutes

Nutritional Value (per serving):

- Calories: 400
- Protein: 35g Calcium: 150mg and Fiber: 5g

Ingredients:
- 4 oz cod fillet
- 1 cup cherry tomatoes
- 1 cup broccoli florets
- 1 tbsp olive oil
- 1 tbsp lemon juice
- 1 tsp garlic powder
- Salt and pepper to taste

Preparation Method:

1. Preheat oven to 375°F (190°C).
2. Place cod fillet on a baking sheet.
3. Toss cherry tomatoes and broccoli with olive oil, lemon juice, garlic powder, salt, and pepper.
4. Arrange vegetables around the cod.
5. Bake for 20 minutes.

Cooking Time: **25 minutes**

Nutritional Value (per serving):
- Calories: 300
- Protein: 25g
- Calcium: 60mg
- Fiber: 6g

Lentil and Spinach Curry

Ingredients:

- 1 cup lentils, rinsed
- 2 cups spinach
- 1 cup diced tomatoes
- 1 cup coconut milk
- 1 onion, diced
- 2 garlic cloves, minced
- 1 tbsp curry powder
- 1 tbsp olive oil
- Salt and pepper to taste

Preparation Method:

1. Heat olive oil in a pot over medium heat.
2. Sauté onion and garlic until tender, about 5 minutes.
3. Add lentils, tomatoes, coconut milk, and curry powder.
4. Bring to a boil, then reduce heat and simmer for 25 minutes.
5. Stir in spinach and cook until wilted.
6. Season with salt and pepper.

Cooking Time: 35 minutes

Nutritional Value (per serving):
- Calories: 350
- Protein: 15g
- Calcium: 100mg and Fiber: 15g

Baked Chicken Parmesan

Ingredients:

- 4 oz chicken breast, breaded
- 1/2 cup marinara sauce
- 1/4 cup mozzarella cheese, shredded
- 1/4 cup Parmesan cheese, grated
- 1 tbsp olive oil
- 1 tsp Italian seasoning
- Salt and pepper to taste

Preparation Method:

1. Preheat oven to 375°F (190°C).
2. Place breaded chicken breast on a baking sheet.
3. Drizzle with olive oil and season with Italian seasoning, salt, and pepper.
4. Bake for 20 minutes.
5. Top with marinara sauce and cheeses, and bake for another 10 minutes.

Cooking Time: 30 minutes

Nutritional Value (per serving):

- Calories: 400
- Protein: 35g
- Calcium: 250mg
- Fiber: 4g

Ingredients:

- 1 cup chickpeas, cooked
- 2 cups spinach
- 1 cup diced tomatoes
- 1 cup vegetable broth
- 1 onion, diced
- 2 garlic cloves, minced
- 1 tbsp olive oil
- 1 tsp cumin
- Salt and pepper to taste

Preparation Method:

1. Heat olive oil in a pot over medium heat.
2. Sauté onion and garlic until tender, about 5 minutes.
3. Add chickpeas, tomatoes, vegetable broth, and cumin.
4. Bring to a boil, then reduce heat and simmer for 20 minutes.
5. Stir in spinach and cook until wilted.
6. Season with salt and pepper.

Cooking Time: 30 minutes

Nutritional Value (per serving):

- Calories: 300
- Protein: 12g
- Calcium: 100mg and Fiber: 10g

Spaghetti Squash with Tomato Basil Sauce

Ingredients:
- 1 spaghetti squash
- 2 cups diced tomatoes
- 1/4 cup fresh basil, chopped
- 1/4 cup Parmesan cheese, grated
- 2 garlic cloves, minced
- 1 tbsp olive oil
- Salt and pepper to taste

Preparation Method:

1. Preheat oven to 375°F (190°C).
2. Cut spaghetti squash in half, remove seeds, and place cut-side down on a baking sheet.
3. Bake for 40 minutes.
4. Heat olive oil in a skillet, sauté garlic for 1 minute.
5. Add tomatoes and cook until softened, about 10 minutes.
6. Scrape spaghetti squash strands into a bowl, top with tomato sauce, basil, and Parmesan.

Cooking Time: 50 minutes

Nutritional Value (per serving):
- Calories: 250
- Protein: 8g, Calcium: 150mg and Fiber: 6g

Ingredients:

- 1/2 cup quinoa, cooked
- 1 cup grilled vegetables (zucchini, bell peppers, eggplant)
- 1/4 cup feta cheese, crumbled
- 1 tbsp olive oil
- 1 tbsp lemon juice
- Salt and pepper to taste

Preparation Method:

1. Grill vegetables until tender, about 10 minutes.
2. Combine quinoa, grilled vegetables, and feta cheese in a bowl.
3. Drizzle with olive oil and lemon juice.
4. Season with salt and pepper.

Cooking Time: 20 minutes

Nutritional Value (per serving):

- Calories: 350
- Protein: 12g
- Calcium: 150mg
- Fiber: 6g

Baked Eggplant Parmesan

Ingredients:
- 1 eggplant, sliced
- 1 cup marinara sauce
- 1/2 cup mozzarella cheese, shredded
- 1/4 cup Parmesan cheese, grated
- 1 tbsp olive oil
- 1 tsp Italian seasoning
- Salt and pepper to taste

Preparation Method:

1. Preheat oven to 375°F (190°C).
2. Arrange eggplant slices on a baking sheet, drizzle with olive oil, and season with Italian seasoning, salt, and pepper.
3. Bake for 20 minutes.
4. Top with marinara sauce and cheeses, and bake for another 10 minutes.

Cooking Time: 30 minutes

Nutritional Value (per serving):
- Calories: 350
- Protein: 15g
- Calcium: 250mg
- Fiber: 8g

Tofu and Vegetable Stir-Fry

Ingredients:
- 4 oz firm tofu, cubed
- 1 cup broccoli florets
- 1/2 cup bell peppers, sliced
- 1/2 cup snap peas
- 1 tbsp soy sauce
- 1 tbsp olive oil
- 1 garlic clove, minced
- 1 tsp ginger, minced

Preparation Method:

1. Heat olive oil in a skillet over medium-high heat.
2. Add garlic and ginger, sauté for 1 minute.
3. Add tofu and cook until browned, about 5 minutes.
4. Add vegetables and soy sauce, and stir-fry until tender, about 5 minutes.

Cooking Time: 15 minutes

Nutritional Value (per serving):
- Calories: 250
- Protein: 15g
- Calcium: 200mg
- Fiber: 5g

Baked Chicken and Sweet Potato

Ingredients:

- 4 oz chicken breast
- 1 medium sweet potato, diced
- 1 tbsp olive oil
- 1 tsp paprika
- 1 tsp garlic powder
- Salt and pepper to taste

Preparation Method:

1. Preheat oven to 375°F (190°C).
2. Place chicken and sweet potatoes on a baking sheet.
3. Drizzle with olive oil and season with paprika, garlic powder, salt, and pepper.
4. Bake for 25 minutes.

Cooking Time: 30 minutes

Nutritional Value (per serving):

- Calories: 400
- Protein: 30g
- Calcium: 60mg
- Fiber: 6g

Greek Yogurt Parfait

Ingredients:
- 1 cup Greek yogurt
- 1/2 cup mixed berries
- 1/4 cup granola
- 1 tbsp honey

Preparation Method:

1. Layer Greek yogurt, mixed berries, and granola in a glass.
2. Drizzle with honey on top.

Cooking Time: 5 minutes

Nutritional Value (per serving):
- Calories: 250
- Protein: 15g
- Calcium: 200mg
- Fiber: 4g

Apple and Almond Butter

Ingredients:
- 1 medium apple, sliced
- 2 tbsp almond butter

Preparation Method:

1. Slice the apple into wedges.
2. Serve with almond butter for dipping.

Cooking Time: 5 minutes

Nutritional Value (per serving):
- Calories: 200
- Protein: 4g
- Calcium: 80mg
- Fiber: 5g

Ingredients:
- 1/2 cup hummus
- 1 carrot, cut into sticks
- 1 cucumber, cut into sticks
- 1 bell pepper, sliced

Preparation Method:

1. Arrange the veggie sticks on a plate.
2. Serve with hummus for dipping.

Cooking Time: 5 minutes

Nutritional Value (per serving):
- Calories: 150
- Protein: 5g
- Calcium: 40mg
- Fiber: 6g

Ingredients:
- 1/4 cup chia seeds
- 1 cup almond milk
- 1 tbsp honey
- 1/2 tsp vanilla extract

Preparation Method:

1. Combine chia seeds, almond milk, honey, and vanilla extract in a bowl.
2. Mix well and refrigerate for at least 4 hours or overnight.

Cooking Time: 5 minutes (plus refrigeration)

Nutritional Value (per serving):
- Calories: 200
- Protein: 5g
- Calcium: 200mg
- Fiber: 10g

Banana Oat Cookies

Ingredients:
- 2 ripe bananas
- 1 cup rolled oats
- 1/4 cup dark chocolate chips

Preparation Method:

1. Preheat oven to 350°F (175°C).
2. Mash bananas in a bowl.
3. Mix in rolled oats and dark chocolate chips.
4. Drop spoonfuls onto a baking sheet.
5. Bake for 15 minutes.

Cooking Time: 20 minutes

Nutritional Value (per serving):
- Calories: 150
- Protein: 3g
- Calcium: 20mg
- Fiber: 4g

Trail Mix

Ingredients:
- 1/4 cup almonds
- 1/4 cup walnuts
- 1/4 cup dried cranberries
- 1/4 cup dark chocolate chips

Preparation Method:
1. Mix all ingredients in a bowl.

Cooking Time: 5 minutes

Nutritional Value (per serving):
- Calories: 200
- Protein: 4g
- Calcium: 30mg
- Fiber: 3g

Cottage Cheese and Pineapple

Ingredients:
- 1 cup cottage cheese
- 1/2 cup pineapple chunks

Preparation Method:
1. Mix cottage cheese and pineapple chunks in a bowl.

Cooking Time: 5 minutes

Nutritional Value (per serving):
- Calories: 180
- Protein: 15g
- Calcium: 150mg
- Fiber: 2g

Avocado Toast

Ingredients:
- 1 slice whole-grain bread
- 1/2 avocado
- 1/4 tsp sea salt
- 1/4 tsp black pepper

Preparation Method:

1. Toast the bread.
2. Mash avocado and spread on toast.
3. Season with sea salt and black pepper.

Cooking Time: 5 minutes

Nutritional Value (per serving):
- Calories: 200
- Protein: 4g
- Calcium: 20mg
- Fiber: 6g

Edamame

Ingredients:
- 1 cup edamame, shelled
- 1/4 tsp sea salt

Preparation Method:

1. Boil edamame in salted water for 5 minutes.
2. Drain and sprinkle with sea salt.

Cooking Time: 10 minutes

Nutritional Value (per serving):
- Calories: 150
- Protein: 12g
- Calcium: 60mg
- Fiber: 8g

Smoothie Bowl

Ingredients:
- 1 banana
- 1/2 cup frozen berries
- 1/2 cup Greek yogurt
- 1/2 cup almond milk
- 1 tbsp chia seeds

Preparation Method:

1. Blend banana, frozen berries, Greek yogurt, and almond milk until smooth.
2. Pour into a bowl and top with chia seeds.

Cooking Time: 5 minutes

Nutritional Value (per serving):
- Calories: 250
- Protein: 10g
- Calcium: 200mg
- Fiber: 7g

Dark Chocolate and Almonds

Ingredients:
- 1 oz dark chocolate
- 1/4 cup almonds

Preparation Method:

1. Serve dark chocolate with almonds.

Cooking Time: 5 minutes

Nutritional Value (per serving):
- Calories: 200
- Protein: 4g
- Calcium: 40mg
- Fiber: 5g

Ingredients:
- 1 cup cherry tomatoes
- 1/2 cup mozzarella balls
- 1/4 cup fresh basil leaves
- 1 tbsp balsamic glaze

Preparation Method:

1. Thread cherry tomatoes, mozzarella balls, and basil leaves onto skewers.
2. Drizzle with balsamic glaze.

Cooking Time: 10 minutes

Nutritional Value (per serving):
- Calories: 150
- Protein: 8g
- Calcium: 200mg
- Fiber: 2g

Roasted Chickpeas

Ingredients:
- 1 cup chickpeas, cooked
- 1 tbsp olive oil
- 1 tsp paprika
- 1/2 tsp garlic powder
- Salt to taste

Preparation Method:

1. Preheat oven to 400°F (200°C).
2. Toss chickpeas with olive oil, paprika, garlic powder, and salt.
3. Spread on a baking sheet and roast for 20 minutes.

Cooking Time: 25 minutes

Nutritional Value (per serving):
- Calories: 180
- Protein: 8g
- Calcium: 60mg
- Fiber: 6g

Cucumber and Hummus Bites

Ingredients:
- 1 cucumber, sliced
- 1/2 cup hummus

Preparation Method:

1. Slice the cucumber into rounds.
2. Top each slice with a spoonful of hummus.

Cooking Time: 5 minutes

Nutritional Value (per serving):
- Calories: 100
- Protein: 4g
- Calcium: 30mg
- Fiber: 3g

Berry and Nut Mix

Ingredients:
- 1/4 cup dried blueberries
- 1/4 cup dried cherries
- 1/4 cup almonds
- 1/4 cup walnuts

Preparation Method:

1. Mix all ingredients in a bowl.

Cooking Time: 5 minutes

Nutritional Value (per serving):
- Calories: 200
- Protein: 4g
- Calcium: 50mg
- Fiber: 4g

Dessert:

Greek Yogurt Berry Tart

Ingredients:
- 1 cup Greek yogurt
- 1 cup mixed berries
- 1 tbsp honey
- 1 pre-made graham cracker crust

Preparation Method:

1. Spread Greek yogurt evenly in the graham cracker crust.
2. Top with mixed berries and drizzle with honey.
3. Chill for 30 minutes before serving.

Cooking Time: 30 minutes (chilling time)

Nutritional Value (per serving):
- Calories: 200
- Protein: 8g
- Calcium: 150mg
- Fiber: 3g

Chia Seed Pudding

Ingredients:
- 1/4 cup chia seeds
- 1 cup almond milk
- 1 tbsp honey
- 1/2 tsp vanilla extract

Preparation Method:

1. Combine chia seeds, almond milk, honey, and vanilla extract in a bowl.
2. Stir well and refrigerate for at least 4 hours or overnight.

Cooking Time: 5 minutes (plus refrigeration time)

Nutritional Value (per serving):
- Calories: 180
- Protein: 5g
- Calcium: 200mg
- Fiber: 10g

Ingredients:
- 2 large apples
- 2 tbsp honey
- 1 tsp cinnamon
- 1/4 cup chopped walnuts

Preparation Method:

1. Preheat oven to 350°F (175°C).
2. Core the apples and place them in a baking dish.
3. Fill the centers with honey, cinnamon, and chopped walnuts.
4. Bake for 25 minutes.

Cooking Time: 30 minutes

Nutritional Value (per serving):
- Calories: 150
- Protein: 2g
- Calcium: 20mg
- Fiber: 4g

Avocado Chocolate Mousse

Ingredients:

- 1 ripe avocado
- 2 tbsp cocoa powder
- 2 tbsp honey
- 1/4 cup almond milk
- 1 tsp vanilla extract

Preparation Method:

1. Blend all ingredients until smooth.
2. Refrigerate for 30 minutes before serving.

Cooking Time: 5 minutes (plus refrigeration time)

Nutritional Value (per serving):

- Calories: 200
- Protein: 2g
- Calcium: 30mg
- Fiber: 6g

Lemon Ricotta Cheesecake

Ingredients:
- 1 cup ricotta cheese
- 1/2 cup Greek yogurt
- 1/4 cup honey
- 2 eggs
- 1 tsp lemon zest
- 1 tsp vanilla extract

Preparation Method:

1. Preheat oven to 350°F (175°C).
2. Mix ricotta cheese, Greek yogurt, honey, eggs, lemon zest, and vanilla extract until smooth.
3. Pour into a greased baking dish.
4. Bake for 30 minutes.

Cooking Time: 35 minutes

Nutritional Value (per serving):
- Calories: 250
- Protein: 12g
- Calcium: 200mg
- Fiber: 0g

Ingredients:
- 2 ripe bananas, mashed
- 1 cup blueberries
- 1/2 cup almond flour
- 1/4 cup oats
- 1/4 cup honey
- 2 eggs
- 1 tsp baking powder
- 1 tsp vanilla extract

Preparation Method:

1. Preheat oven to 350°F (175°C).
2. Mix all ingredients until well combined.
3. Pour into a greased loaf pan.
4. Bake for 45 minutes.

Cooking Time: 50 minutes

Nutritional Value (per serving):
- Calories: 200
- Protein: 5g
- Calcium: 50mg
- Fiber: 4g

Almond Flour Cookies

Ingredients:
- 1 cup almond flour
- 1/4 cup honey
- 1/4 cup coconut oil
- 1 tsp vanilla extract
- 1/4 tsp baking soda

Preparation Method:

1. Preheat oven to 350°F (175°C).
2. Mix all ingredients until well combined.
3. Drop spoonfuls onto a baking sheet.
4. Bake for 12-15 minutes.

Cooking Time: 20 minutes

Nutritional Value (per serving):
- Calories: 150
- Protein: 3g
- Calcium: 30mg
- Fiber: 2g

Pumpkin Chia Seed Pudding

Ingredients:
- 1/4 cup chia seeds
- 1 cup almond milk
- 1/4 cup pumpkin puree
- 1 tbsp maple syrup
- 1/2 tsp cinnamon

Preparation Method:

1. Combine all ingredients in a bowl and stir well.
2. Refrigerate for at least 4 hours or overnight.

Cooking Time: 5 minutes (plus refrigeration time)

Nutritional Value (per serving):
- Calories: 180
- Protein: 5g
- Calcium: 200mg
- Fiber: 10g

Baked Pears with Honey and Almonds

Ingredients:
- 2 pears, halved and cored
- 2 tbsp honey
- 1/4 cup sliced almonds
- 1/2 tsp cinnamon

Preparation Method:

1. Preheat oven to 350°F (175°C).
2. Place pear halves in a baking dish.
3. Drizzle with honey, and sprinkle with sliced almonds and cinnamon.
4. Bake for 20 minutes.

Cooking Time: 25 minutes

Nutritional Value (per serving):
- Calories: 150
- Protein: 2g
- Calcium: 20mg
- Fiber: 4g

Dark Chocolate Avocado Brownies

Ingredients:

- 1 ripe avocado
- 1/2 cup dark chocolate chips, melted
- 1/2 cup almond flour
- 1/4 cup cocoa powder
- 1/4 cup honey
- 2 eggs
- 1 tsp vanilla extract
- 1/2 tsp baking soda

Preparation Method:

1. Preheat oven to 350°F (175°C).
2. Blend avocado until smooth.
3. Mix in melted dark chocolate, almond flour, cocoa powder, honey, eggs, vanilla extract, and baking soda.
4. Pour into a greased baking dish.
5. Bake for 25 minutes.

Cooking Time: 30 minutes

Nutritional Value (per serving):

- Calories: 200
- Protein: 4g
- Calcium: 30mg
- Fiber: 5g

Yogurt and Berry Popsicles

Ingredients:
- 1 cup Greek yogurt
- 1 cup mixed berries
- 2 tbsp honey

Preparation Method:

1. Blend Greek yogurt, mixed berries, and honey until smooth.
2. Pour into popsicle molds and freeze for at least 4 hours.

Cooking Time: 5 minutes (plus freezing time)

Nutritional Value (per serving):
- Calories: 100
- Protein: 5g
- Calcium: 100mg
- Fiber: 2g

Ingredients:
- 1 cup rolled oats
- 1/2 cup almond flour
- 1/4 cup honey
- 1/4 cup coconut oil
- 1/4 cup raisins
- 1 egg
- 1 tsp vanilla extract
- 1/2 tsp baking soda

Preparation Method:

1. Preheat oven to 350°F (175°C).
2. Mix all ingredients until well combined.
3. Drop spoonfuls onto a baking sheet.
4. Bake for 12-15 minutes.

Cooking Time: 20 minutes

Nutritional Value (per serving):
- Calories: 150
- Protein: 3g
- Calcium: 30mg
- Fiber: 2g

Ingredients:
- 1 cup strawberries, halved
- 1 cup blueberries
- 1 cup pineapple chunks
- 1 cup kiwi, sliced
- 2 tbsp honey
- 1 tbsp lime juice

Preparation Method:

1. Combine all fruits in a large bowl.
2. Mix honey and lime juice in a small bowl, then drizzle over the fruit.
3. Toss gently to combine.

Cooking Time: **10 minutes**

Nutritional Value (per serving):
- Calories: 150
- Protein: 2g
- Calcium: 50mg
- Fiber: 4g

Ingredients:

- 2 cups shredded coconut
- 1/2 cup honey
- 2 egg whites
- 1 tsp vanilla extract

Preparation Method:

1. Preheat oven to 325°F (165°C).
2. Mix all ingredients until well combined.
3. Drop spoonfuls onto a baking sheet.
4. Bake for 15-20 minutes.

Cooking Time: 25 minutes

Nutritional Value (per serving):

- Calories: 150
- Protein: 2g
- Calcium: 10mg
- Fiber: 3g

Mango Coconut Chia Pudding

Ingredients:
- 1/4 cup chia seeds
- 1 cup coconut milk
- 1/2 cup mango puree
- 1 tbsp honey

Preparation Method:

1. Combine chia seeds, coconut milk, and honey in a bowl and stir well.
2. Refrigerate for at least 4 hours or overnight.
3. Layer with mango puree before serving.

Cooking Time: 5 minutes (plus refrigeration time)

Nutritional Value (per serving):
- Calories: 200
- Protein: 4g
- Calcium: 40mg
- Fiber: 8g

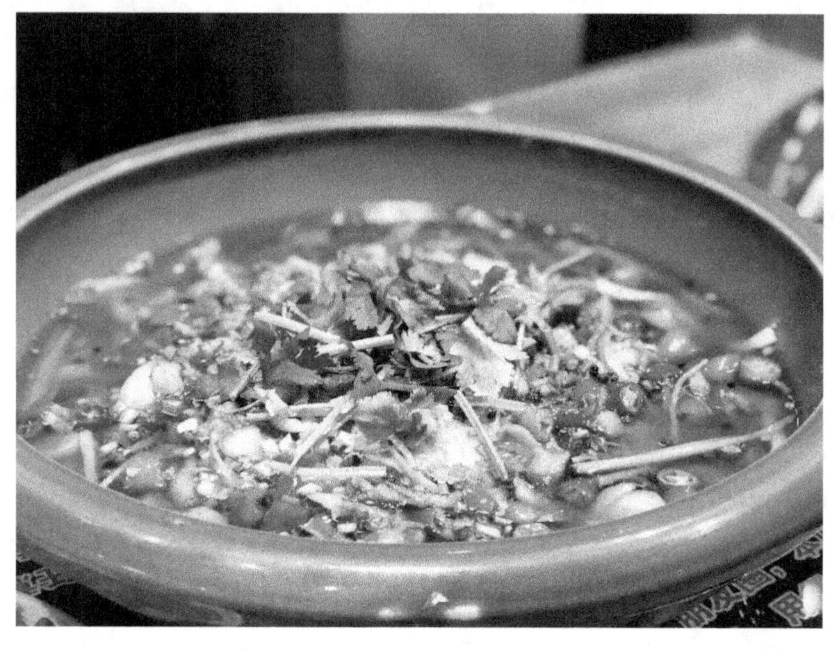

As we reach the conclusion of the "Osteoporosis Diet Cookbook for Women," it's essential to reflect on the profound journey you've embarked upon. This collection of recipes is more than just a guide to nutritious and flavorful meals; it's a testament to the power of mindful eating and the incredible impact it can have on your health and well-being.

Osteoporosis can be a daunting diagnosis, but it's important to remember that you are not alone, and there are effective ways to combat and manage this condition. By choosing foods that are rich in calcium, vitamin D, and other essential nutrients, you are taking significant steps toward strengthening your bones and improving your overall health. Each recipe in this book has been crafted with care, focusing on the vital nutrients needed to support bone density and reduce inflammation.

But this cookbook is about more than just nutrition. It's about empowerment and reclaiming control over your health. It's about finding joy in the kitchen and discovering new flavors and combinations that nourish both your body and soul. It's about creating a lifestyle that embraces wellness and supports long-term health.

To every woman reading this, know that your health journey is uniquely yours, and every step you take toward better nutrition is a victory. The recipes in this book are tools to help you, but the real change comes from within you. Believe in your strength and resilience. Embrace this dietary shift not as a restriction but as a celebration of what your body needs and deserves.

As you close this book, remember that every meal is an opportunity to nurture yourself. Let this be the beginning of a vibrant, healthful, and fulfilling chapter in your life. Your commitment to adopting and adapting to this osteoporosis-friendly diet is a powerful act of self-love and dedication to your future. Here's to stronger bones, better health, and a brighter tomorrow. You've got this.

Weekly Planner

Monday

Tuesday

Wednesday

Thursday

Friday

Saturday

Sunday

Weekly Planner

Monday

Tuesday

Wednesday

Thursday

Friday

Saturday

Sunday

Weekly Planner

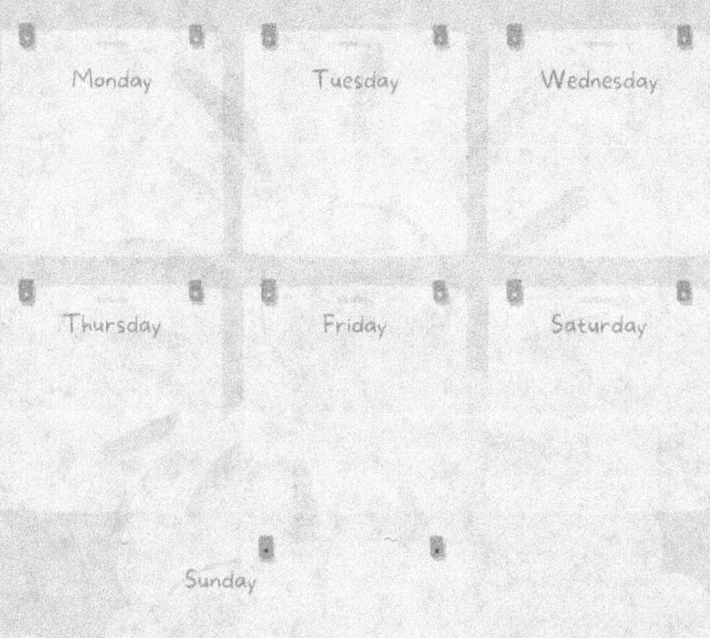

Weekly Planner

Monday

Tuesday

Wednesday

Thursday

Friday

Saturday

Sunday

Weekly Planner

Monday	Tuesday	Wednesday
Thursday	Friday	Saturday
Sunday		

Weekly Planner

Monday

Tuesday

Wednesday

Thursday

Friday

Saturday

Sunday

Weekly Planner

Monday

Tuesday

Wednesday

Thursday

Friday

Saturday

Sunday

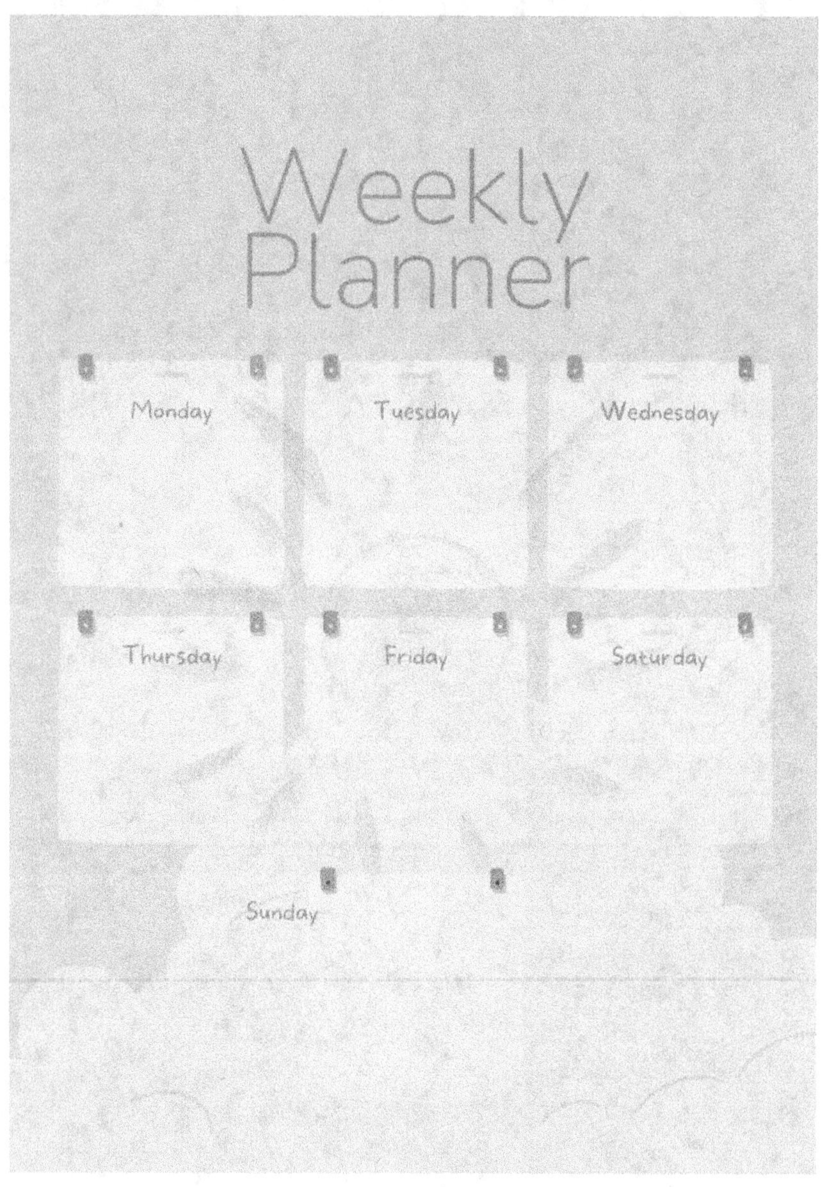

Weekly
Planner
Monday
Tuesday
Wednesday
Thursday
Friday
Saturday
Sunday

Weekly Planner

Monday

Tuesday

Wednesday

Thursday

Friday

Saturday

Sunday

Weekly Planner

Monday

Tuesday

Wednesday

Thursday

Friday

Saturday

Sunday

Weekly Planner

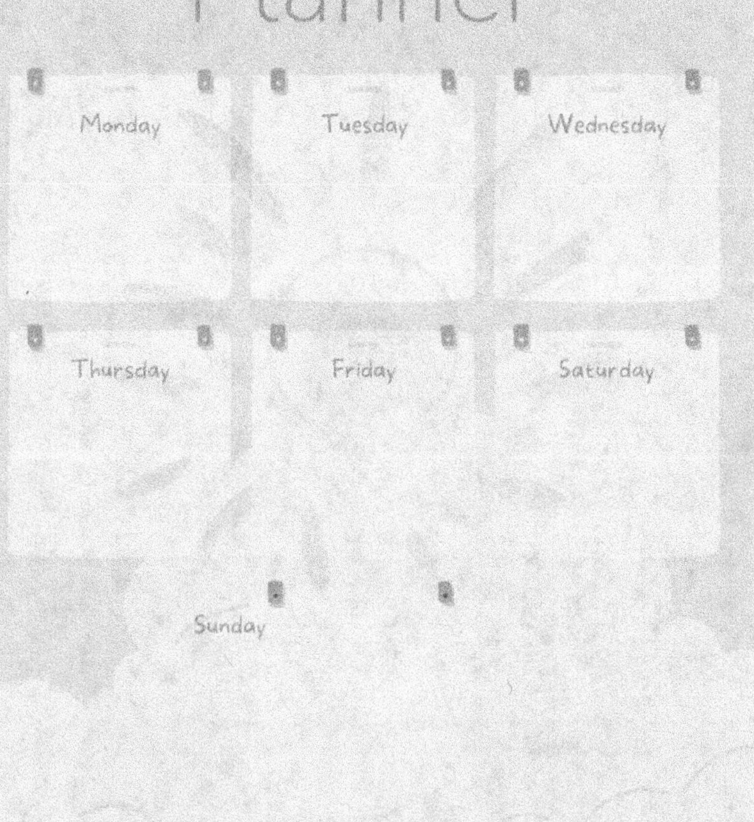

Weekly Planner

Monday

Tuesday

Wednesday

Thursday

Friday

Saturday

Sunday

Weekly Planner

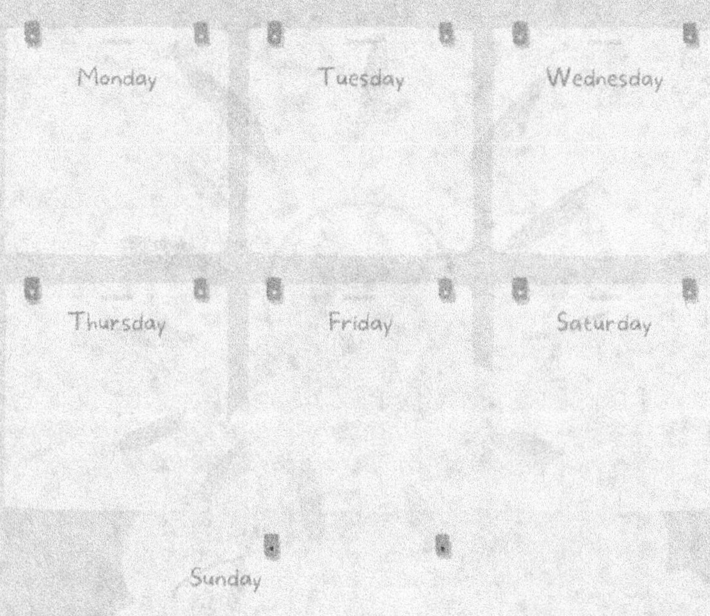

Weekly Planner

Monday

Tuesday

Wednesday

Thursday

Friday

Saturday

Sunday